Willpower

----- ⊷⊷⊷⊶ -----

The Ultimate Guide To Unlocking Spartan Self Discipline And Shifting To A Success Mindset

By Curtis Leone

Table of Contents

The information herein is offered for informational purposes solely, and is universal as so. The presentation of the information is without contract or any type of guarantee assurance.

The trademarks that are used are without any consent, and the publication of the trademark is without permission or backing by the trademark owner. All trademarks and brands within this book are for clarifying purposes only and are the owned by the owners themselves, not affiliated with this document.

Introduction

Congratulations on taking the first step towards unlocking Spartan self-discipline and shifting to a Success Mindset! Maybe you've already begun your journey of self improvement, maybe this is your first step on that journey; regardless of where you are in life there is always room for improvement!

This book will focus on learning ways to improve your life from a civilization that is still studied to this day, the mighty Spartans, and shifting your point of view from a negative or average one, to a powerful Success Mindset.

The Spartans of Greece were legendary for their perseverance and steadfastness in the face of seemingly insurmountable odds. The proper assessment of and adaptation to their environment, their rigid commitment to military excellence, and the exultation of personal austerity every Spartan upheld secured this ancient civilization a place in the history books as a culture to emulate.

The self-discipline practiced by each and every Spartan both on the battlefield and in their daily lives was a truly powerful way of living. With your mastery of Spartan self-discipline you too will come to possess the unconquerable Success Mindset, becoming the living legend of your own life!

Introduction

Although often downplayed in personal development plans, confidence is a vital factor to success. You need a certain degree of confidence in anything you do, from cultivating rewarding personal relationships to reaching the highest professional goals. The confidence of each Spartan in not only themselves, but in the Spartan standing at his side on the battlefield was paramount to their success. Believing in yourself is the first step to having others believe in you.

Sadly, exuding confidence is easier said than done. Many people struggle to summon the confidence they need to succeed, and it can severely impact their perceived quality of life. While a lack of confidence can sometimes be due to distinct clinical reasons such as depression or anxiety, many of us often simply feel unable to live up to society's standards.

Whether that means attaining an ideal look and body weight, or learning to overcome failure, building up your self-esteem can seem like the most difficult task, but it is by no means impossible. Any individual, no matter how helpless they may feel at times, has the power within them to turn things around in their favor.

The Spartans became eligible for their legendary army at the age of 20, but their life expectancy averaged around 35. Today's life expectancy in the United States is around 82, so if you're reading this book before the age of 47, you'd still be in training! And even if you're in your 60s, you'd still be a greenhorn with a lot to learn.

The Spartan army never stopped evolving and adapting to its environment; this is a key component of the Success Mindset. This path to personal improvement requires that you keep an open mind to new ideas and perspectives, and that you never sell yourself short! No one is perfect and all of us have our demons to battle in life, but each and every one of us has the right to make the best of what we have.

This book contains insight and strategies that will allow you to reshape your sense of self-worth, see yourself in a new, positive light, and build up the confidence you need to tackle any hurdle life may throw your way. What this book does not contain is a list of miraculous life-changing tricks.

The Spartans' success on the battlefield was not achieved through some divine intervention or magical devices; the sweat, blood, and effort of warriors bought their victories. In the same way, your daily perseverance will be what ultimately leads to your success.

Most of the things you will read here will seem like common sense once you think about it, but that's often the case when our self-esteem is down - things that may seem so natural to others somehow manage to completely elude our judgment. Once you've shifted into the Success Mindset, these concepts will become second nature.

The first step to building confidence requires that you do something that sounds easy, but that's actually rather hard to do for most of us, and that is to consider and understand your real flaws and weaknesses. Mastery of their terrain led to many victories for the Spartans.

Mastery comes from understanding, and while you may not need to find the best mountain pass to establish a foothold in, you will need to firmly establish yourself by acknowledging and accounting for your flaws. Fortunately, there's a silver lining here - your flaws are very likely not as bad as you think they are.

Introduction

When our confidence is down, we tend to be way too harsh on ourselves, and judge ourselves unrealistically. A pessimistic attitude colors your perception of everything, including yourself. A Success Mindset does not come from a lack of flaws, but from a realistic assessment of our challenges and the perseverance to overcome them.

The second stop on our way to success is the most exciting, because it involves taking action. That means switching from a passive role in your own life to taking on a more active role. Spartan youth entered into the *agoge* system at age 7, training daily until the age of 20, at which point they moved into adult Spartan life, a life of continued systems and rules.

Interestingly, our actions serve to reinforce our mindset, so projecting more confidence can strengthen our faith in our own abilities over time. In other words, small actions undertaken each day will help to gradually build up your sense of self-worth. As your sense of self-worth continues to improve, the daily "chores" you suffer will become daily "tasks" you undertake to perpetuate your Success Mindset.

Spartan self-discipline kept its men ready for battle in an ever-tumultuous time. It will take you diligently sticking to your daily goals if you are to be ready for everything life throws at you; being the best you that you can be every day will ensure that the best you is fighting your daily battles!

The third chapter is similar to the first one, but instead of realizing your faults, it asks you to realistically evaluate your strengths. Once you've learned your terrain, it's time to learn your weapons! The Spartans famed military strength was upheld by men wielding the best instruments they could fashion to the best of their abilities.

Battle formations and tactics were developed and implemented by leaders, but when it came to winning battles, the Spartan soldier's self-discipline in training with his spear and his shield decided who lived and who died that day.

By now you've probably noticed a pattern - building confidence demands a lot of introspection and (sometimes difficult) soul-searching. The well of power that you will have to drink from if you are to become the best you that you can be has to come from within you! If you're wondering why this is mentioned third, the reasoning behind it is simply that most people with low self-esteem are unaware of their strengths.

Sadly, many of us think we do not have any strengths at all, but this couldn't be farther from the truth! Every Spartan had his or her place in society, and equality was a concept perpetuated by focusing on the strengths of the individual. Taking action each day allows us to discover the things we are actually good at, and to learn how we can use them to our advantage. This empowerment of self will be paramount in the solidifying of your Success Mindset moving forward.

And lastly, our final chapter covers the notion of tracking progress as you advance on your journey of self-discovery and improvement. It is important to be able to look back and see how far you're come, all that you've achieved and how you have changed for the better. But it can be quite tricky to do, because these changes are largely mental and emotional, so they are not as easily quantifiable as becoming fit or other physical changes.

There are, however, a few interesting tips to track the many subtle ways in which you have improved over time, and seeing those tangible improvements can help you further strengthen your confidence. The Spartan self-discipline you will have

Introduction

achieved will have opened your eyes to so many of life's joys that you may have once considered unattainable.

You may even find yourself laughing at how easily you've achieved the heights you once considered impossible.

The Success Mindset you will enjoy will not only be helping you to overcome life's obstacles, it will be lending even more pleasure to the beauty that life has to offer. This final chapter will teach you how to stop and smell the roses along the way, and catalogue their beauty for the future.

Before we start, it's important to keep in mind that being confident does not equate with being arrogant or vain. The point is not to feel superior to everyone else, but to understand yourself and learn how to become the best version of you that you can be, so that you can achieve the personal and professional goals that you have set for yourself.

Spartan self-discipline and a Success Mindset are personal endeavors; measuring yourself against someone else, even positively, is not the goal.

Chapter 1:

Understanding Your Flaws

When we perceive ourselves in a negative light, naming our flaws seems like the easiest of things. Off the top of our heads, we're able to list an array of perceived issues that degrade our self-image, such as the following five:

"I'm overweight / ugly."

"I can't get a job."

"I never get promoted at work."

"I can't attract a date."

"I'll never have a spouse/children."

Although these kinds of negative thoughts plague many people at some point or another, none of them represent faults that cannot be overcome. In fact, most of the flaws we think we have are not our real flaws at all, they're just a matter of skewed self-perception. When we think so poorly of ourselves, we're undermining our chances of succeeding in what we set out to achieve and we're perpetuating a seemingly inescapable vicious circle of negative reinforcement.

Chapter 1: Understanding Your Flaws

In psychology, this way of thinking is regarded as a defense mechanism that allows us to victimize ourselves and escape responsibility for our problems, and it works like this:

"I cannot succeed in what I set out to do so it must mean I am decisively flawed in a way that is out of my control."

In truth, by thinking this way you are simply avoiding to admit that you've been sabotaging yourself all along and that you've relinquished control over what you do with your life. But if you were to re-evaluate yourself from a fresh perspective, the five flaws we listed before would look something like this:

"I tend to overeat and neglect my hygiene and fitness."

"I don't perform well at job interviews."

"I don't try to compete with my colleagues at work."

"I wait for potential dates to approach me."

"I'm afraid of intimacy / commitment."

While these statements refer to the very same problems we mentioned at the beginning of this chapter, the main difference this time around is that you've recognized that the source of your misfortune resides in your way of thinking rather than some unbeatable deficiency. This approach helps shift your mindset from feeling helpless to feeling empowered and capable of dealing with your problems in a constructive way. They are not insurmountable issues that will stop you in your track forever, but mere hurdles that can eventually be overcome.

Consider the Spartan army at the battle of Thermopylae, the famous scene of the 300 Spartans who took on the million man Persian army of Xerxes I. The odds were overwhelmingly stacked against the Greeks defending their homeland from invasion. The seemingly obvious choice was to surrender the land; retreat and survive to attempt a counterattack. Thermopylae, however, was one of two main access routes for the Persian Empire's vast army to advance into Greece. Leaders agreed that Artemisium and Thermopylae had to stand for the Greek army's strategy to succeed.

The Spartan army, knowing that they absolutely had to stop the waves of Persians crashing upon their shores, chose the battleground which they would hold: the narrow coastal pass known as "The Hot Gates".

Instead of thinking:

"Their numbers are far too great, there's simply no way we can hold them."

The Spartans thought:

"We must control the terrain to best optimize our manpower if victory is to be achieved."

The Spartan king's decision of where to take on Xerxes and his Persian army was a realistic, accurate, and impactful assessment that made all the difference in the effectiveness of his soldiers. Funneling the seemingly endless Persians into the narrow pass, the Spartans decimated their enemy's ranks. The daily devotion and discipline of the Spartans hardened its soldiers into the premier military of the age. The Spartans held their last line for two full days of battle against odds that numbered a hundred to one. Finally, a traitor from Sparta revealed the location of a small shepherd's path that allowed Xerxes to slip a small number of Persians behind the Spartan line, flanking them, and ending their legendary stand.

While they ultimately suffered a defeat at Thermopylae, the time that King Leonidas's Spartans bought the rest of the Greek army, as well as the casualties they inflicted upon the Persians, were direct causes of Xerxes' withdrawal from Greece, and the routing of the rest of the Persian invasion the following year. It was not the resounding victory the Greeks thought they needed, but the Spartans' defeat was not without its value, and the same is true of your flaws.

Everyone has shortcomings, everyone loses battles, but with a Success Mindset you learn to focus on the bigger picture: winning the war!

The beginnings of a Success Mindset are the removal of the negativity from your attitude, and the shifting towards a more neutral realism. The early stages of this shift do not ask you to jump straight into optimism yet. The Spartan example of a tactical defeat should inspire you to remember that wars can still be won even when battles are lost.

Things may not always go your way, but if you continue to do your absolute best the tides will eventually shift in your favor. Shifting from negativity to realism will allow you to begin laying the blocks in the foundation of a Success Mindset that, when paired with Spartan self-discipline, will ultimately lead you to grow from realism to optimism.

At this point you might be asking yourself how you can keep your self-assessment realistic if your perception of who you are is so negative. Well, the answer is that, as with all things, you must start small. Instead of focusing on all of your failures at once and allowing yourself to crumble under their weight, try looking at each issue individually and rationalize how you could improve it.

By funneling the Persians into a narrow pass that suppressed their numbers into man-to-man pairings, the Spartans were able to maximize the effectiveness of their individual soldiers. Take on your problems on a case-by-case basis. What actions can be taken to realistically help your situation, and is a change in approach necessary?

As it turns out, if you keep thinking the way you've always thought, you'll keep getting the same results you always got. Any meaningful improvement starts from within, with a change of mindset. Again, the shift to a Success Mindset cannot and will not happen all at once. It is said that a journey of a thousand miles begins with the first step. This is a powerful message, but it should be noted that this journey is only completed by subsequent steps after that.

Unless you take that first step onto a jet, you won't find yourself at the end of that journey by the end of the day, or even by the end of the week! Your journey of life will be a series of steps taken incrementally, but with a Success Mindset and Spartan self-discipline both your journey and your destination will be rewarding and enjoyable. It all begins by changing your mindset!

To understand how to do this, let's take the five issues we've already listed throughout this chapter as examples of how to engage in constructive self-assessment. The first one is extremely common and it deals with feeling ugly and unattractive. In the more realistic assessment, the feeling is still there, but now you're not blaming your situation on some external factor out of your control, such as luck, fate or genetics.

Instead you're taking responsibility for your body and recognizing that you may not have the best diet. A poor diet and overeating can be symptoms of underlying emotional problems that you may not even be consciously aware of, which is why it can feel like they're not in your power to change. Scientists are now suggesting that eating too much and finding gratification in food shares many of the characteristics of drug addiction, effectively locking the brain in a destructive feedback loop. Body image issues can also lead people to neglect their hygiene and fitness (for example to not shave or shower as much as someone with a higher self esteem) as they feel it wouldn't make a difference anyway.

In reality, neglecting to take care of your body is what perpetuates a negative body image in the first place. By making positive changes to your hygiene routine, you will start to see an improvement in your overall appearance, which will in turn encourage you to continue taking better care of yourself. This is one of those "chores" that will become "tasks" once you begin to look at things in the new light of a Success Mindset.

A Spartan's dedication to his military craft was daily. They knew that at any time they may be called upon to defend their homes. You won't be asked to pick up your spear and shield and fight to defend your home, but you may need to bring your best smile to a job interview at a moment's notice. If you are brushing your teeth two or more times a day, flossing, and generally making sure your dental health is in order, you will have more confidence when you have to sit across the desk from a potential employer.

Humans are creatures of habit; changing your life will be a matter of changing your habits. Assess your daily habits. Do you take care of your personal hygiene the way you should? If not, why do you think that is? Are those valid reasons not to take care of yourself? Of course not! These smallest flaws are the easiest to correct. If you forget to brush your teeth before getting into bed, get out and do it! Don't let yourself talk yourself out of it! You'll find yourself replacing bad habits before you know it!

The second and third statements both refer to confidence and success in the professional field. If you are unable to draw a potential employer's interest in you, although you were called in for an interview, it's clear that your resume and qualifications are not the problem. Maybe it's down to how you perform at the actual job interview.

Appearing more confident and agreeable will leave a stronger impression and significantly improve your chances of landing the job you want. Here's where the Spartan self-discipline will pay off; your daily devotion to improving your appearance, health, and overall mental well-being will make you a more attractive candidate for whatever position you seek.

Similarly, if you're aiming for a promotion but it seems impossible to actually get it, it's likely that you haven't shown a strong enough interest for your employer to notice, or that you've allowed your colleagues to steal all of your employer's attention. Once the Success Mindset starts taking root, however, you will begin to command the respect and appreciation you deserve.

In both situations, the solution requires a change in perspective and action, and an effort to understand your real weakness (which can be worked with), rather than resigning and blaming it all on an insurmountable, fictitious one. If you are unable to get the job or promotion you seek, consider whether you have underperformed, or whether you lack the confidence to pursue your goals with determination. Remember, whatever flaws you find in your character or performance are not set in stone.

The shift to the Success Mindset will open your eyes to solutions for all of your problems; it will take determination on your part to take the steps necessary to better yourself. It is often not enough to simply wait around for a job or a promotion, you must confidently and actively carve out opportunities for yourself. For example, you should try to approach each job interview with confidence in your abilities, and seek out promotion opportunities even if your boss isn't explicitly laying them down before you.

The Spartans were not known for living an easy or lavish life; theirs was a life of rigorous adherence to strict policies of austerity and military training regiments, but when it came to conquering their enemies they were unrivaled.

The last two issues we mentioned relate to one's personal life, their ability to attract and keep a romantic partner, and to form a family. In the first scenario, the person feels unable to attract a potential date, which means they are always waiting to be approached by others rather than try to approach someone themselves.

Similar to the case of the person waiting for their boss to consider them for a promotion, when you are waiting to be asked out you're inadvertently passing up on countless date opportunities because you lack the confidence to ask someone out yourself. The principal culprit for this type of hesitation is the fear of rejection. Some people feel that rejection would deepen the negative feelings they already have about themselves, but at the end of the day, not taking a chance at all is functionally indistinguishable from rejection. This means not that you're unable to get a date, but that you're actually afraid to take a chance, effectively standing in your own way.

The fear of rejection is a perfectly normal condition, but a Success Mindset is not the mindset of a normal person! The shift to a Success Mindset will help you realize all you have to offer, and you will soon realize that rejection by another person does determine your self worth. Once you are becoming the best you that you can be, anyone would be lucky to share your life!

It's also important to look at this realistically - if you start asking people out, it is very likely that you will, sooner or later, experience rejection. But this should not discourage you from trying again with someone else. Sometimes people simply do not click, the chemistry or communication just isn't there.

It does not mean that everyone you approach will react in a similar fashion, and again, it is not a reflection of your worth! It is important to keep trying and not let one rejection drag you down, because trying is by default more desirable than never trying at all. The Spartans faced odds that no other army would have faced, and even in defeat they succeeded in turning the tide of the war.

The more that you unlock and adhere to Spartan self-discipline, the better and better you will become, and you will become more and more confident in your Success Mindset. You will soon find yourself so excited for the opportunities your new life-style opens up that a little rejection will hardly spoil the all the fun you're having!

Chapter 1: Understanding Your Flaws

The benefits of understanding your flaws will become more and more apparent the more realistic you are about them. There is no character flaw so grave that it cannot be overcome by one of the strengths you are gifted with. Do not get discouraged if you find yourself in need of a lot of work. Be excited at the huge difference a little time and effort is going to make in your life! The path you will soon be walking will not be the easiest, but it will be the most rewarding experience of your life.

In fact, the path you will be walking will *be* a rewarding life, because the Success Mindset is not a destination, but a journey. Just think, if you accidentally cultivated these flaws, how much more powerful will your strengths be when you're applying yourself with Spartan self-discipline? You are more than capable to getting yourself over that hump of resistance that has been mocking you for months!

Chapter 2:

Taking Action Each Day

Once you've taken the time to understand your faults and you have framed them in such a way that allows you to tackle them constructively, you might be wondering how to proceed next. How do you begin to take the actual steps necessary to build your confidence up, where do you start?

The answer depends on a case-by-case basis, but one commonality is that you must find your own personal *motivation* to become confident. In other words, it is important to start working on fulfilling your goals. The area for your Success Mindset has been surveyed, it's time to start building the foundation!

The Spartans were not always a culture focused on military strength and the austerity of its citizens. At first Sparta was just a small village on the bank of a river, not much different from any other village on the bank of a river. Then, in the mid 8th Century BC, during a period of unparalleled strife and lawlessness, a semi-mythical king and lawmaker emerged name Lycurgus who would change the values of their society, setting in motion the gears, which would turn Sparta into a household name.

Chapter 2: Taking Action Each Day

His focus was on three main virtues: equality among citizens, austerity, and military strength. He founded the *agoge*, a rigorous training and education program that began transforming young Spartans from age seven. The program trained the Spartan population in hunting, dancing, singing, communication arts, stealth, military training—including pain tolerance—and cultivated loyalty to the Spartan group.

Sparta then fought wars to secure their foothold in the region, growing into a large city-state of Greece that controlled most of the Peloponnesus. Their success can be directly attributed to their military power and the self-discipline of their citizens who adhered to training throughout their entire lives. It is this Spartan self-discipline that you will use to keep yourself ready to take on any and all challenges life throws at you.

At this point, you might be feeling discouraged enough by past failures that you are not even willing to try. After all, you've been down this road before, and it has only led to disappointment. If this is how you feel, think carefully about *how* you used to do things before, when you wanted to pursue a specific goal.

Consider that the problem wasn't the goal itself or your lack of ability to ever achieve it, but that you simply went about it the wrong way at the time. Remember to accurately assess the flaw that may have hindered you in the past, and come up with a new solution to your problem.

For example, if your goal is to get a better job or to land the promotion you desire, it's a good idea to start by taking small steps that improve your odds and make you a better, more desirable candidate. Instead of immediately shooting for the moon and setting yourself up for failure, take the time to prepare yourself so that when the time is right, you are ready to face that challenge.

Maybe you need to work on building a more impressive resume or to go above and beyond at your current job to make your employer take note of your performance. Whatever you find to be the area you need to work on, just remember that you are more powerful than your flaws. At 20, Spartan men in the *agoge* officially entered into the Spartan military, and were expected to enlist into one of the public messes.

They had to be voted in unanimously, and rejection was common for average soldiers. The best and brightest competed for spots in the *hippeis*, the royal guard, with the rest having to hone themselves to the absolute best of their abilities to make it into a public mess by age 30. If it was achieved, a Spartan man then became a citizen and only then could he marry, vote, or hold public office.

The grueling task was by no means easy, but the rewards were inclusion in one of the most respected societies of ancient times, and were well worth the effort! It should be noted that even these most elite of warriors sometimes took up to a decade to achieve the position they desired, so don't lose heart!

If your goal is of a more personal nature, say you're trying to find a suitable partner for marriage, think of the ways you've deal with it in the past. Perhaps you proposed too soon or maybe you started a relationship with a person who was not interested in such a commitment in the first place? If so, then you might have saved yourself from heartache later down the line with a more realistic assessment.

Chapter 2: Taking Action Each Day

A Success Mindset is all about being realistic first, optimistic second. This is a classic example of how being overly optimistic can create unrealistic expectations, which can lead to disastrous and disappointing results. You ultimately only have control over yourself, finding the best partner will become easiest when you find yourself to be the best you that you can be. Your positivity will be rooted in the reality of the effort that you are putting into yourself.

That kind of positivity resonates within positive people, and you will find yourself engaging with more and more of the kind of people you genuinely relate with, because you will be more and more true to yourself. This will open all kinds of doors to relationships with people with whom you genuinely connect, and the fruits of these relationships will be much sweeter.

Even if commitment isn't your end-goal, or the goal of the person you find yourself attracting, you may end up finding a soul mate and changing both of your minds together. The possibilities are endless in life, and a Success Mindset will unlock the doors to so many beautiful ones for you.

The key to working towards your goals is understanding that it is a slow process that requires dedication, and often, even personal sacrifice. Unfortunately, there is no magical, quick way to success, it's all about persevering with small actions taken each day, that build upon what you have already achieved. Improving personal hygiene is a huge first step for the Success Mindset. A hygienic self is a healthy self, and a healthy self is a happy self.

Make sure to take care of these littlest of things first and foremost. As insignificant as it may seem to get yourself out of bed to brush the teeth you forgot to, it is a small correction of a flaw that you can accomplish with just the slightest willpower.

Bigger challenges will inevitably arise, and as they say, practice makes perfect.

Practice overcoming the small obstacles, and you will get a form down for when the larger ones arise. If you are impatient, try to rush things or won't stay committed to your goals, chances are very high that you will never accomplish them. So if you've set the goal of brushing your teeth before bedtime every night, don't make any excuses! Get it done! Realistically assess how you spend your time in life, set realistic timetables for yourself, but also allow yourself time to breathe! If you set daily goals for yourself and you accomplish them, don't push too hard; enjoy your success and relax knowing that you've earned it.

You will quickly discover that you're able to love yourself more, and that you're much more appreciative of what you have achieved, when you feel that you have truly *earned* your keep. Indeed, an important part of building up your self-esteem is valuing yourself realistically and knowing that your success is in your own hands.

The first step in finding your motivation is to set goals for yourself. Sometimes, when your self-esteem is down and you feel lost, you can also experience a crippling feeling of aimlessness. You might feel like you don't know what you want to do with your life, that things don't make sense or that you're generally apathetic.

But in reality, even if you are not fully conscious of your goals yet, if you've looked inward, analyzed yourself and have made efforts to understand your faults, it means you have thought about the things you want from life and why you haven't got them yet. So on some level, you *do* have goals or at least a general idea of what your goals could be. Now it's time to reaffirm them clearly, and consciously realize the type of person you want to become.

As we've previously established, progress is not made in leaps, but with steady, daily actions. These actions may each seem of little significance at first glance, but if you consider them together, they form the building blocks of your new-found self-confidence. A good idea here is to set small milestones for yourself - realistic things that can be realized in a relatively short span of time.

Again, consider your personal hygiene. Once your personal hygiene habits become perfect, how about making the bed every morning? Starting your day by doing something productive, and doing it well, is a great way to make sure that the rest of your day has firm ground to stand on.

Let's take physical fitness as another example - should one of your goals be to improve your appearance and become healthier, you might find yourself wanting to lose a few pounds. Assuming you want to shed quite a bit of weight and you settle on a specific amount (say 20 - 30 pounds), you need to consider that weight loss is a slow process that can take months or even years to produce healthy, sustainable results. Sadly, many dieters are impatient and wish to see results quick, so they become unmotivated within a few weeks or even days if those results do not appear.

A very common pitfall of dieting is giving up too soon simply because you fixated on the end goal too much. Remember though, you're shifting to a Success Mindset. The time required to see results may be months, but what are a couple of months when compared to the rest of your life? Once you form healthy habits, you will find yourself enjoying multiple benefits that will spur you on to continue the path to success.

Two important aspects to take into consideration when trying to lose weight is that it's a lengthy process that requires long term commitment, and that the rate at which we lose weight is not equally reliable for all people. For example, if one person is able to lose 2 pounds per week, this process may be slower or faster for someone else. It's also good to keep in mind that your own weight loss rate can fluctuate - during some weeks you might find that you lose less weight than during other weeks.

Just keep in mind that while weight loss is the goal, the ultimate goal is to live healthier and to be happier. Take the time to appreciate the beauty of the area you go jogging in. If you go to a gym, use your time there meditate on your life and re-focus yourself on your goals outside of fitness. Whatever you do, try to squeeze every last ounce of positivity and beauty that you can out of it; this is a true exercise of the Success Mindset.

Another commonly overlooked detail is that if you work out to lose weight, you will be replacing some of the adipose tissue you lose with muscle tissue. So when you weigh or measure yourself, it may not immediately look like you lost enough fat, but remember to keep in mind the reality of the situation: the changes are happening even if you can't see them yet.

Don't let what you perceive to be true, stop you from remembering the actual truth, which is that with Spartan self-discipline and adherence to hard work. You will reach your goals. Similarly, if your goal is to enhance your strength and muscle tone, you may be tempted to constantly check how much you are able to lift week on week, although you might not be making consistent gains each week. The key to remember is that you're on the right path. If everything magically changed all at once, what else would you do?

Chapter 2: Taking Action Each Day

A great life is not a destination, it is a journey! When you take care of your health, mental and physical, you live a better life, and that's the whole point! The exercise, the hygiene habits, making the bed, all of these activities will go from dreaded "chores" to "tasks" on a daily checklist that can be checked off, cataloguing your success.

With respect to personal relationships, you can start by setting the seemingly modest goal of meeting new people. Many individuals with low self-esteem experience social anxiety that prevents them from approaching others or from engaging in positive social activities. If you are finding yourself in a similar situation, then the simplest way to start being more social is to just put yourself out there, even if you're not immediately successful.

You will find that when you begin to work on yourself, you will have more confidence when meeting new people. Once you like being around yourself more, you will find more reasons to believe that other people may do the same. A Success Mindset, even in its early forms, is attractive; people are drawn to people who are working on themselves. So get out there!

Try to talk to people, and say hello when you meet someone you like. You don't have to be obviously flirty or wear a sign that says you're looking for a date, just be yourself and you might find that most people tend to respond positively when approached in an affable manner. Remember, exude that Success Mindset! Instead of focusing on appearing friendly to potential romantic partners only, try to make this your default attitude with all the new people you meet.

Friends are an important part of life, sometimes even more so than romantic partners. Finding friends who are also on roads of self-improvement can be hugely beneficial to your efforts as well as theirs. Another thing you can do is to start up a cordial conversation with a stranger in a public place, such as at the mall. They don't need to be a romantic interest, but doing so will help build up your confidence in approaching new people. Make sure you pick inoffensive topics of general interest and don't be discouraged if it doesn't always go as well as you'd like.

The person you picked might not have expected a conversation or they may be dealing with their own social insecurity issues. Enroll in art or music classes at adult education centers, visit your local library and find book clubs that might interest you, find a bar with music you like and become a regular; there are a million ways and places to meet new people, find one that suits your lifestyle!

Once you've built up enough confidence to deal with social situations, you might want to consider approaching people you would like to date. Maybe one of your friends has a friend that you've come to admire. Take a chance! As we've established in the last chapter, actively trying is infinitely preferable to doing nothing, even though you must be emotionally prepared for rejection too. To reiterate, we all experience rejection at some point in life, it's all just part of the great dating game and it doesn't mean that you are less valuable as a person or chronically incapable of finding the partner of your dreams. It's like they always say, if at first you don't succeed, try and try again!

When you do manage to get a date, it's important to think well about how you want to proceed. Sealing the date means you made a good first impression, but it doesn't mean you've got it in the bag. It make take several dates to assess whether you really are compatible with that person, and it helps if both of you are true to each other and to yourselves.

It might be tempting to put on a mask that you think might make you appear more desirable, but in reality it's not who you are and your partner will be able to tell eventually as your relationship develops. The goal is to be far enough along in your Success Mindset that you no longer feel the need or desire to wear a mask. Once you have set upon the path to the best you that you can be, you'll want someone to walk that path with you. Your partner can't help you achieve the best you that you can be if your partner doesn't know the real you, or the you that you want to be!

If you find yourself dating someone who is beginning to look incompatible, don't sabotage your progression by lying to yourself or to that person. It's better to move on with your life, and let them move on with theirs. There's a saying that goes, "Sometimes you have to kiss a few frogs to find your prince." If the experience of finding a soul-mate is so rare, then realistically speaking that means that there are going to be A LOT of people out there who just aren't for you, no matter how badly you want them to be.

A good relationship won't be without its share of work, but it should never feel forced. If you keep that Spartan self-discipline and continue to better yourself daily, and you keep your Success Mindset focused on continuing to better yourself, you will eventually find yourself with the right partner to help actualize your maximum potential.

When you finally are in a long-term relationship, you might discover that you still experience insecurity and doubts about your future. Setting small milestones and building up your confidence is just as important at this stage as it was before. The Success Mindset is like a garden: even though you have beautiful flowers blooming you still have to pluck the weeds.

Maybe you are unsure about how committed both of you are or if you're on the same wavelength with regards to what you want from life and your shared future. Mutual trust and communication are the cornerstones of a relationship, so make sure you talk to your loved one each day and don't let any conflicts, no matter how small, go by unresolved. These things can add up over time and negatively impact your relationship goals in the long run.

This is where you will have to rely on your Spartan self-discipline: you absolutely MUST remain honest with yourself and your partner. Keep the lines of communication open and honest. Approach every negative situation with the intent of resolving the matter peacefully; don't focus on who's to blame, focus on how to move forward.

If you're ready to propose to your partner, test the waters first, making sure that they too are ready for such an important step in your relationship. Some people are so focused on their careers that the idea of a family may even come as a surprise. Your relationship goals will likely vary, but if you keep communication open and honest, you can find middle ground with each other.

Each couple has its own particularities, and in your case, it might be preferable to keep discussing the matter openly over a period of time than to simply pop the question to an unsuspecting partner. If they aren't open to the idea at first, give them time. If they continue to be closed to the idea, and your end-goals become very apparently different, move on to find someone who shares your end-goals. Remember, stay real!

Don't waste your time wearing a mask. Finding the right person for you will require you to call upon that Spartan self-discipline to keep yourself focused on the right path for your life. When you do find the right person, and the relationship is built on truth and self-improvement, you will discover that feeling like you have a strong, real bond with your partner bolsters your self-esteem, your positivity and your faith in the future.

Us humans are gregarious creatures and our sense of self-worth is strongly linked to the success of our social bonds. If you find the right person, and get married, keep building on your marriage with small gestures each day; you will eventually find yourself ready to discuss having children as well.

As your positivity snowballs and your partner's positivity snowballs, the idea of creating new little snowballs of positivity will be attractive to you both, and you'll be ready to face the challenges of parenthood with a smile, strong resolve, and the loving help of a committed partner.

Our final point touches on your professional goals. Like most of us, you might be driven by a desire to grow your career and feel like your skills and hard work are being rewarded accordingly. The Success Mindset you cultivate will yearn to share your talents with the world. Just like with losing weight, an important factor to success is acknowledging from the get go that you can't "cheat" the system or take short cuts to earn you that sought-after promotion.

The most reliable course of action is to work steadily and consistently on improving your credentials and affirming yourself at your place of employ. Again, the Spartan self-discipline is not a magical super-occasion; it is a continued devotion to small, daily exercises of growth. You have to learn to crawl before you walk, and walk before you run. Don't get discouraged at first, eventually, if you stick to it, you'll find yourself running marathons!

Another useful tip is to cultivate positive relationships with your colleagues and your superiors. If everyone in the office is talking about the big game on Friday, maybe you should watch it, even if you have no real interest in sports. Sports are the modern way for men and women to peacefully let out aggression, and they cultivate healthy competition between rivals.

You don't have to absolutely lose your identity in the crowd, or become a hardcore sports fan, but it never hurts to take interest in a new hobby, especially when the people you work with share that hobby. Maybe it's not sports, maybe it's a genre of music that a lot of your coworkers enjoy. Broaden your horizons a little and it can go a long way. The human aspect can be just as important in helping you secure a promotion as your credentials.

Don't forget that an office is a social space and a friendly and likable attitude can considerably improve your career prospects. That small talk about the game on Friday or last week's concert can make you feel more accepted. And remember those hygiene tips! Keeping your personal appearance fresh never hurts your chances!

In case you're self-employed or trying to get a start-up rolling, try to focus on careful planning before doing anything else. It's easy to get overwhelmed, but at the core of every start up there is ultimately a product, which needs to be marketed and sold. You want to make sure you have a clear idea of what you want to achieve, and then try pitching it to friends and acquaintances to see how it might be received. Is your product necessary?

If it's not necessary, is it exciting or engaging in some other way? Use your Success Mindset to look realistically at your project. Researching the market can help you establish whether there's a demand for it, and working diligently on all of the small details will help to improve your chances of success. Just like with everything else we discussed, entrepreneurship doesn't happen overnight, it takes a lot of preparation, learning, as well as trial and error, to get everything right.

Research business plans online to help you formulate your own, learn all of the factors you will have to account for when you get your business started, even the ones you'll have to make sure to take care of on the road to getting your business off the ground. Whatever you set out to achieve, try not to lose heart at the first hurdle and you will see that the more you are able to persevere, the better your confidence is and the better you feel about yourself. The Spartans' preparation for war was what made them such a force to be reckoned with. They ate, breathed, and slept warfare; they were always prepared.

You won't find yourself being called to battle a million man army any time soon, but eating, breathing, and sleeping ideas of the Success Mindset (realistic assessments, achievable goals, perseverance in the face of adversity) will keep you ready to face anything life has to throw at you with the fortitude of a legendary warrior.

Chapter 3:

Discovering Your Strengths

If you've taken note of the advice we offered in the previous 2 chapters, it means that you now understand why you failed your goals in the past, and that you've started taking daily actions to course-correct.

Have you had to get out of bed to brush your teeth yet? Did you do it? You better have! Your level of confidence should already be on the rise, and even if you haven't yet reached your goals, you know that you're working hard towards achieving them.

But chances are you've also started experiencing some setbacks that are having the opposite effect on you, gnawing away at your newly built confidence. Maybe new flaws are coming to light after you thought you'd eliminated them all.

If this is where you are right now, then it's time to learn how to deal with mistakes and disappointment in a positive way, turning them into learning experiences rather than failures. Remember the Spartans; even a losing battle can win the war!

The reason why you needed to first understand your faults and take constructive action that built up confidence, is that when you really lack self-confidence and you're rife with self doubt, you are unable to discern what you're good at. People with a crippling low self-esteem are not capable of accurately appreciating their strengths.

It is only after you've accomplished some of the things you strive for (even if they were small accomplishments) that you're able to uncover your abilities and skills. Bear in mind that these are likely things you've had your entire life, you just haven't had the chance to put them to good use yet, or to fully reap their benefits. One of the focuses for training in the *agoge* was poetry.

Consider poetry; it is comprised of the same words in the same language that we use every day, but when used in a more considered manner these ordinary words become pieces of beautiful works of art.

You possess many personality attributes that you might not even consider as strengths. But in your day-to-day life, in your career and even in your intimate relationships, they may prove to be invaluable assets to long-term success. Some of these traits are:

- Loyalty

- Kindness / altruism

- A sense of duty

- Perseverance

- Adaptability

- Intelligence / Creativity

- Patience

...And the list goes on. A good idea would be to sit down and jot the strengths that you feel have revealed themselves to you thus far throughout your journey to build up your confidence. Remember, being realistic is key to the Success Mindset. By now you've been improving your daily life, be realistic about how much you've improved!

Think about the ways you've benefited from your strengths, how they've helped you take on your daily actions, or how they've helped improve your social and professional skills. Paying special attention to the way your strengths have helped you is an invaluable tactic in solidifying your self-esteem, as it will re-affirm the notion that you have intrinsic value as a human being, regardless of any hardship you've had to endure.

Your past failures were hurdles along your path, but they by no means define who you are. Your strengths and actions do! The more confident you become in realizing your strengths, the more you will project an image of self-assurance and self-reliance that your peers and loved ones will also be able to notice.

You will thus have entered a positive feedback loop - the more favorable everyone's attitude toward you becomes, the more it encourages you to love and value yourself and the more opportunities will reveal themselves to you. This is the awesome power of the Success Mindset: the more you benefit from it, the more positivity it generates in others, and the more it comes back to benefit you again!

Let's take a look at how a simple trait like loyalty can completely shape the way other people see you. You may be tempted to think it hasn't served you well in the past because you've allowed other people to take advantage of your loyalty and use it to hurt you.

Chapter 3: Discovering Your Strengths

While it is true that there are people out there who will always try to exploit your strengths and use them against you, your loyalty makes you invaluable both on a personal and on a professional level.

It generally means that you are an excellent friend, a trustworthy partner that is in for the long haul, and a serious, dependable employee that your superiors can always count on. Loyalty is like the mighty Spartan shield, the *aspis*! This piece of equipment was absolutely indispensible to a Spartan warrior.

The *aspis* was designed over many years of bashing and shield-wall formation training to not only protect the Spartan wielding it, but to protect the phalanx formation as a whole. It was so important to the Spartan's battle formation that death was a preferable option to losing it in battle.

Your loyalty is a strength that lends the might of your strength to your entire company, whether it's professional or personal, and is a highly sought after trait by employers and potential mates alike. A Spartan would release his sword or spear before releasing his shield; never let loyalty to the wrong person make you feel like you should be less loyal!

A Success Mindset solution to the betrayal of loyalty would be to realistically assess the situation, which found you misplacing your loyalty. Were there signs that your trust was being broken?

Maybe you did not see them in time *this time*, but with Spartan self-discipline towards correcting your flaws, you *will* catch them next time, before they spell disaster again. Just remember to keep in mind that loyalty *is a strength* and don't take on the responsibility of the flaws if someone betrays that loyalty.

Kindness and altruism are attributes that pretty much speak for themselves. Some of the daily actions you take could revolve around doing good and spreading positivity around you. But again, just like in the case of loyalty, they may sadly seem like weaknesses if you let other people take advantage of you.

Don't ever let anyone make you feel like your kindness is a flaw, because genuine kindness can be rare and it's arguably one of the most uplifting human traits. It can impress, touch and inspire others on another level, trumping even creativity and intelligence. Kindness and altruism are important traits that not only feel good to you, but also have the power to influence those around you for the better.

If you're tempted to think that using kindness as leverage makes you selfish, consider that at the end of the day, it's a win-win for all parties involved - it helps bolster your self-respect and it makes the world a better place. Kindness and altruism are like the *xiphos* blade or *dory* spear in the hands of a Spartan.

Wield them with effectiveness, and you will find yourself the toast of your company. The Spartans did not fight with brutish weapons like the axe or mace; their weapons required finesse and dedication to a martial art.

If kindness is already inherent to your persona, lucky you! Most have to train very hard in the art of meeting negativity with a smile to ever reach any level of effectiveness. If you find you have a knack for being a positive person, you can hone this skill to take you very far in life.

Positivity you share with others always comes back to you, and being positive in your daily life is the stepping stone to take your Success Mindset's realism to the next step: optimism! Unchecked optimism in the wrong mindset can be dangerous, but someone with a Success Mindset who learns to look on the realistically brighter side of life is a truly powerful person indeed.

A sense of duty makes you a partner everyone can trust, whether it is in marriage or in your career. It ties in to your sense of loyalty, and it means that you are able to take things very seriously when the situation calls for it. Some specific career prospects make it a point of how important duty can be (such as the military, law enforcement or emergency services), but no matter what career path you choose, we can guarantee that any serious employer will treasure your dependability.

Every Spartan was trained in the *agoge* to cultivate loyalty to the Spartan culture. Your sense of duty can help in unlocking your Spartan self-discipline: if you are to make the most impact for your group, you must be devoted to becoming the best you that you can be!

The importance of perseverance is especially obvious when trying to build up a confident mindset, and it is an indispensable ingredient to success in any long-term goals. Remember, a Success Mindset is not born of a lack of flaws, it is the realistic assessment of life's challenges and the perseverance to overcome them! It means that you are at least willing to brave any setbacks, even if you don't readily know how to tackle them and correct your mistakes.

It is best described as your willingness to press on. For example, even the fact that you are reading this book right now is an expression of your perseverance, as it implies you have not given up on trying to better yourself as a person and become more confident. But being perseverant does not mean you never doubt yourself, or that nothing can slow you down or even stop you in your tracks.

It simply means you don't want to give up and are ready to start over even after things have gone badly. This concept is quite possibly the most important aspect of the Success Mindset. Perseverance is the little voice in your head that says "Get up! Try again! How about we do it like this instead this time?"

If you don't already possess perseverance, don't worry, it's achievable! How? By doing! When life gets you down, when you fail, don't give up! In soccer, coaches often yell out "FOLLOW UP!" or "FOLLOW THROUGH!" when a player misses a shot on the goal. It means to keep charging the net, even if you realize you've missed the shot.

The ball often times bounces off a rail or the goalie and ends up in a spot where a follow up shot can be taken, but if the player hasn't followed the ball up to the goal, or followed through with his attack, he won't be in position to take that second shot. It takes perseverance to keep going when you initially miss your mark. The opportunity to score will open again, make sure you're always moving towards it!

Adaptability is a valuable trait because it means that you are naturally a survivor. You've dealt with failures in the past, but have not allowed them to break your spirit. You also know that those were not the last times life was challenging you. There will always be new challenges, perhaps especially so once you start realizing your goals and you find yourself on an upward path.

The old saying "hope for the best, expect the worst" still rings true and it helps tremendously to be mentally prepared to handle any tough challenges that life may throw your way. It does not necessarily mean that these difficult challenges will ever come, but being ready for the worst-case scenario also means that you are able to tackle lesser problems with much more ease.

Adaptability was what set the Spartans apart from their Greek brothers and sisters. The blades they wielded were considerably shorter than other Greek blades of the time, and their shields were bigger. These adaptations made their phalanxes more powerful: their massive shields better protected their men who were able to wield the shorter blades with more effectiveness in the confined spaces.

They adapted the weapons they fought with to suit their specific needs in battle, and the effects of such adaptations are still lauded to this day. Be ever vigilant for ways to renew and adapt new concepts into your Success Mindset. Being the best you that you can be means never settling for "good enough." Life is a continual journey, continue to adapt and improve and you too will achieve paramount success!

The positive steps you've taken since you started following the advice in this book are suggesting that you are much more resourceful than you gave yourself credit for in the past. It's not uncommon to feel stuck, at a loss, or even stupid when your self-esteem is down. But as we've already discussed, these are not realistic self-evaluations, they are just your insecurities speaking for you.

By now you probably have realized that you're intelligent and creative enough to pull yourself up and turn your life around. No matter what some IQ tests suggest, everyone is intelligent enough to succeed in their goals, it's only a matter of using what they have to their advantage. Not everyone possesses equal book smarts and not everyone may be able to become a businessman or a scientist, but those kinds of smarts are not the be all and end all of intelligence.

In fact, research now suggests that there are many other kinds of intelligence that IQ tests and traditional school exams can't even properly test for, but they are attributes that will come to your aid in your day-to-day life. For example, maybe you have a high degree of emotional intelligence and are able to understand other people and to quickly and accurately respond to their needs.

Maybe you have a particular talent, such as that you are a good cook or a good beautician. No matter what career you have, remember not to look down on yourself or compare yourself to others whose careers you perceive as more successful than your own.

Most often, our perception of the people we negatively compare ourselves to is idealized and not realistic at all. There is a saying: "Everybody is a genius, but if you judge a fish by its ability to climb a tree it will live its whole life believing that it is stupid." If you are not on the same level as someone you know or have heard about, the simple answer is: it doesn't matter! Your life is your own personal journey, and focusing on your strengths is how you should judge your abilities.

You shouldn't say:

"She's better at painting than me, I should focus on coloring with crayons."

Nor should you say:

"I'm better at math than he is, he should only focus on chemistry."

Your conversation on creativity and intelligence should sound more like:

"I'm better at math than I am at art, maybe I should draw as a hobby but pursue a career teaching algebra."

Comparing your intelligence and creativity with another person will, at best, only distract you from the most important part of self-improvement: you! When you find the area that you excel in, don't focus on where others are excelling, except to offer encouragement and support. When you focus your Success Mindset on improving the natural abilities that you already have, you will find yourself far more fulfilled, and the feelings of inadequacy in comparison to others will diminish.

In a famous ancient account an Athenian once asked a Spartan why his *xiphos* blade was so short. The Spartan paused a moment, looking down, and after considering it replied: "It's still long enough to reach your heart."

Your patience ties into your perseverance and it gives you a net advantage in achieving any goals you have set for yourself. It means you are less likely to give up along the way, if significant results don't start appearing right away. It also means you are a considerate spouse and lover, and would make a wonderful parent.

But if you feel like patience is not exactly your strong suit, consider a few ways you can cultivate it further, so that it may benefit you in your quest toward you goals. A good way to reliably develop your patience is to practice delaying gratification - for example if you're an impulse shopper and can't seem to slow down, start thinking twice before making any new purchases and ask yourself if you really need those things.

Patience is also key to the Success Mindset; it is not the lack of action that is the highlight of patience, but rather the appropriate action at the appropriate time. It will truly test your Spartan self-discipline to develop patience, but it is another extremely valuable piece of the Success Mindset puzzle.

So by now, hopefully you've come to realize some of your own strengths, and which areas of strength you need to focus energy on in order to grow. One of the most important parts of Spartan society from which to learn is their strict code of honor. Rage, berserker tendencies, or suicidal recklessness was strictly prohibited in the Spartan army, as such behavior was a detriment to the phalanx at large.

To a Spartan, those who wished to fight *and live* were considered far more valorous than those who rushed into a fight with complete disregard to saving their own life. They believed that a warrior was not to fight enraged, but with a calm determined attitude. What can be taken from this ancient mindset and applied to today's challenges is this: brash action yields less powerful results.

If you get upset at your spouse and lash out in anger, yelling or throwing things, what outcome may be achieved? Maybe you scare or sadden your partner into behaving as you see fit, but would not a more preferable and more honorable solution be to change how they believe they should be? If their actions upset you, and they love you, isn't a solution other than one based on fear or sadness achievable?

Chapter 3: Discovering Your Strengths

A calm conversation about what you feel and about what your partner feels will open the doors to a compromise, and that is the truest victory to be won. Behavior can be modified without the need to intimidate. You probably had different points of view on the matter in question, so bring your points of view to the table, and learn from each other to form a new point of view together.

A relationship is all about compromise, about two becoming one.. The same principle can be true of any confrontation though, personal or professional: a compromise reached through mutual respect and understanding is the absolute best way of moving forward together.

If you find yourself in a fix, take a deep breath and a step back, then use your Success Mindset to realistically assess the situation and you will find the proper solution. A calm determined attitude yields the most positive and lasting results.

Chapter 4:

Tracking Your Progress

If you have diligently followed the strategies laid out in the first three chapters of this book, then it means that you are ready to practice the final point, which is tracking your progress. Are you still getting out of bed to brush your teeth? No? You've made it a habit you remember? Congratulations!

In the introduction, we insisted on the importance of focusing on taking small steps in all our endeavors, rather than simply waiting for a miraculous leap. Remember, the journey of a thousand miles can be broken down into step after step. Just keep putting one foot in front of the other; you'll get there!

We compared building up your self-esteem to losing weight and making muscle gains, highlighting that there are many variables that might make your personal experience unique. Remember not to be comparing yourself to others; the only person you can better is yourself, stay focused! No matter what kind of advice you read in self-help books, there will always be something that you need to do slightly different, some way that you need to tweak and personalize the things you learn, so that you can properly use them to your advantage.

Learn as much as you can from as many sources as you can, a person with a Success Mindset never stops learning.

Chapter 4: Tracking Your Progress

Now, once you have a basic grasp of what you need to do, it turns out that tracking progress is easier than you might think. So many things are easier than you think when you're stuck in a negative mindset. The Success Mindset will open your eyes to how easily life can be lived well, and how much fun it can be too!

As you first start to settle into your new routines, you might want to track your progress on a daily basis, and the more comfortable you become in applying what you have learned, you can start tracking less often - maybe once a week. The daily checklist will start happening mentally, and the positivity that stems from it will become naturally inherent as your Success Mindset and Spartan self-discipline lead you to living a better and better life.

The idea is to go over the major events and interactions that have taken place during the course of the day, and think about whether they were positive or negative, whether you could have done something differently, and whether any of them had an influence on your mindset. You don't need to write all of this down, most of this process can be done in your head at the end of the day, but it helps to keep a diary where you put down any important notes or comments that you might have.

You can keep this diary by your bedside for easy access and so that you don't forget to use it each day. If you find yourself enjoying the activity of writing about your day, carry it with you so you can record events on the go. If you find yourself forgetting to write, attach writing in the diary to one of your new healthy habits, like brushing your teeth at night.

And again, if you find yourself forgetting, do your best to correct the situation as soon as you remember. The more frequently you correct yourself, the sooner you will stop forgetting.

To make tracking even easier, you can decide on a small number of relevant questions that you need to answer on a daily basis. These questions will help you evaluate how your confidence levels evolve over time and what are the things that tend to influence you the most. For example, your daily questions could look something like this:

1. What made me feel less confident today?

2. How did I handle that situation?

3. Did this lack of confidence cause me to make more mistakes?

4. What made me feel more confident today?

5. Did that confidence boost help me towards any achievement today?

6. What faults of flaws have I identified today?

7. What strengths have I identified today?

8. What actions could have I taken today to achieve better results?

9. What actions should I take tomorrow?

The idea is to keep things simple, consistent and easily quantifiable over a longer period of time. If the questions you write are too complicated or require very complex answers, it's less likely that you'll be able to keep an accurate track of how you've changed. The purpose of tracking your progress is to assist you in the often times challenging process of self-analysis.

It also helps to preserve your thoughts and perceptions of events as they happen, because later when you try to revisit them in your head, your memory might have skewed important details. Not to mention, plenty of wonderful things will be happening in your life as you continue to improve it. Having a catalogue of pleasurable memories is a fun thing to revisit from time to time. If you've never written a travel journal when you go on vacation, give it a shot!

You'll be amazed at how just the slightest recording of daily events can transport you back to wherever you were visiting. Re-living a fantastic life is just as rewarding, so keep track of all the fun you're having! It will take your Spartan self-discipline to write *every* day, but it is another one of those easily achievable goals that can lend to feeling positive about the effort you're making.

The more you track your progress and engage in self-analysis, the easier it will become for you to understand and judge yourself realistically. After a while, you might find it is very easy to do, so you won't need to track your progress as often, or you won't feel the need to write it down on paper. Tracking your progress in a diary is not meant to be a life-long process, but simply a way to help ease your transition into a healthier, more confident mindset. Of course, if you find yourself enjoying being able to look back on the memories you may have otherwise forgotten, you may want to continue the habit of keeping that diary.

Although it's not meant to be a permanent step, it's important not to neglect tracking your progress, especially at the beginning of your journey. Your Success Mindset will need all the help you can give it in the beginning stages to make sure it takes root and blossoms. For the first few weeks or even months, you might feel like you always have a lot to write down, especially on not so good days when your confidence has taken a more serious hit or when you feel like you've made a lot of mistakes.

This is where your Spartan self-discipline will shine: make yourself do what you know you need to! Don't be afraid of what this process might reveal to you, although it can seem a bit overwhelming at first, it will definitely become much easier and natural to you as the months roll by. The more you improve your confidence, the less you'll feel like you have to write after a while.

An interesting benefit of tracking your progress is that it reinforces the other 3 steps you're already taking to cultivate your sense of self-worth. It helps you understand your faults easier, decide on what the best actions are to take each day, and uncover your strengths, all within a simple and manageable framework. It really puts that realism aspect of the Success Mindset into perspective when you can read over something after the emotional response to the situation has passed. If you look at the nine questions we listed, you can pretty much break them down into two major categories:

- Questions that track the areas you need to improve

- Questions that track the things you are good at

This kind of two-fold approach helps you have a well-rounded, realistic grasp of who you are, with both flaws and strengths. You can tweak and change up the questions however you like, of course, but it is a good idea to keep this two-fold approach in mind whenever you are tracking your daily progress. And remember to keep your questions simple and to the point.

Austerity, a cornerstone of Spartan society, is defined as "extreme plainness and simplicity of style or appearance." The reason this concept is so important is that when you boil things down to their most basic form, stripping away the unnecessary parts, not only can their usefulness or effectiveness be gauged properly, but the effects of change are far more powerful on them. While you don't have to cut out every frill from your life, when it comes to keeping track of your progress you want to maximize the results your efforts achieve.

Therefore, keeping your questions simple to answer directly will make sure that you don't stump yourself when you go to keep track of yourself. These two categories, areas you need to improve and things you are good at, are the simplest representations of the opposite poles that, when studied, are the guide-rails on your path to self improvement. When you look back on yourself months or even years down the line, these basic things are what will stand out to you the most, while the small, specific details will be lost to time.

It is vital to track your progress and your shortcomings with accurate assessments of both. The Spartans *agoge* system was written about by philosophers and historians who witnessed it because of its powerful beneficial impact on Greek citizens. The Spartan's defeat at Thermopylae was recorded as a way to not only catalogue the events of the time, but to celebrate their indefatigable resolve in the face of certain defeat, literally fighting to the end.

It takes an acknowledgement of both the good and the bad times that Sparta endured to really appreciate this amazing ancient civilization. Similarly, by tracking your strengths and weaknesses, one day you too may be able to lend some wisdom and encouragement to someone else who may be ready to start upon their own road of self-improvement.

One final point that should be remembered: all along the way you should be planning your goals, every one from the smallest to the biggest. This chapter discusses writing down checkpoints for yourself to be able to look back on, but keeping a written planner of your goals that you wish to achieve that day, that week, that month or that year is another important part of a successful life.

Most successful professionals keep a person planner full of appointments, to-do lists, grocery lists, and other general schedule items; you should too! Having a list written of what you have to do can help to keep you from getting overwhelmed, and if you find yourself unable to make everything happen that you want to, it can make sure that important tasks you need to accomplish don't get forgotten by the time you have the time to take care of them.

Again, if you find yourself falling short don't give up hope. Sometimes we dream a bit too big. Learn to realistically assess the amount of time you have during the day and you will find yourself creating more and more realistic goals for yourself. Proper time management is a skill that must be developed like any other skill: with practice, practice, practice!

Conclusion

Thank you again for joining me on this journey!

I hope this book was able to help you learn more about unlocking Spartan self-discipline and shifting to a Success Mindset. These concepts are tools that you will hopefully soon be experiencing the true power of! Your friends and family will be astounded at the progress you make and may even ask where this epic person you've become came from. Tell them you always had it in you to be this amazing, it only took unlocking the awesome potential within yourself to achieve such success!

The next step is to go out there and get yourself a diary to start keeping track of your progress, and start making that progress! Remember to keep your assessments realistic and your will to persevere strong. The road to self-improvement is sometimes difficult, sometimes enjoyable, but it is *always* rewarding, and you deserve to be the best you that you can be!

Finally, if you enjoyed this book, then I'd like to ask you for a favor, would you be kind enough to leave a review for this book on Amazon? It'd be greatly appreciated!

Thank you and good luck!